Motion Is Medicine
Your Prediabetes Reversal Blueprint

Shaquelle Falon Thomas

I0449172

Copyright Page:

TABLE OF CONTENTS

PRELUDE

I'm Shaq, a Registered Kinesiologist who leads women living in discomfort to freedom from chronic pain and chronic illness. Allow me to introduce you to the decisions I made to reverse my prediabetes naturally.

I grew up in the early 2000's where low rise jeans and thinness was a trend. As a chubby girl growing up this was pretty mentally damaging. With that being said, I was off and on dieting for as long as I remember. I tried every diet out there and they'd usually last about 3 days then I'd binge eat and fall back into the unhealthy cycle. The MyFitnessPal app and I had a love-hate relationship.

One spring day back in 2016 I had my annual check-up with the doctor — Never an event I was excited for. The doctor took a look through my blood work and said a few words you don't like to hear coming from a doctor.

"Your A1C levels are high. You are prediabetic".

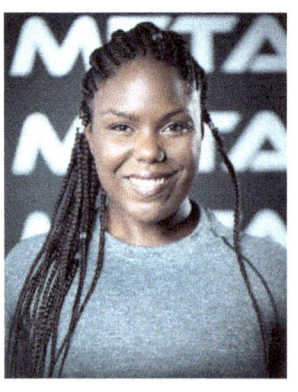

I remember my heart dropping into my stomach because, although I always had my health as a priority in my mind, I never thought I was in a place where pre-diabetes was on my radar.
Now, it's worth mentioning that type 2 diabetes runs in my family big time. If I was being honest with myself, I would have seen

PRELUDE

that I was following the same lifestyle as my family members who have the condition (except they didn't do off-and-on dieting as often as I did).

But still. I was shocked.

After my shock settled in during my checkup; I asked the doctor what I needed to do to reverse the prediabetes. I saw the effects diabetes had on my grandparents' quality of life and I refused to go down that road. I'll give you one guess as to what the doctor said… "lose weight, eat healthy and exercise".

Still to this day this advice has not helped me the way my doctor may have thought it would. I had been told to lose weight and exercise at almost every doctor's visit since I was a child. But, this time I decided to make a lasting change. And I've only been getting healthier since that day. Instead of diving head first into another fad diet; I decided to take it slow by changing my "least healthy" habits one by one.

After about a year I lost over 70lbs and my blood sugar levels were great.

Ever since then I've gradually added new healthy habits into my life when I felt ready to do so. With that being said I've had my ups and downs over the years. But, overall, my healthy habits won the battle.

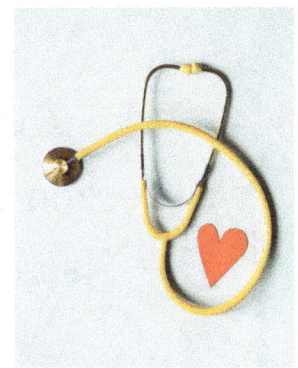

CHAPTER 1: UNDERSTANDING PREDIABETES

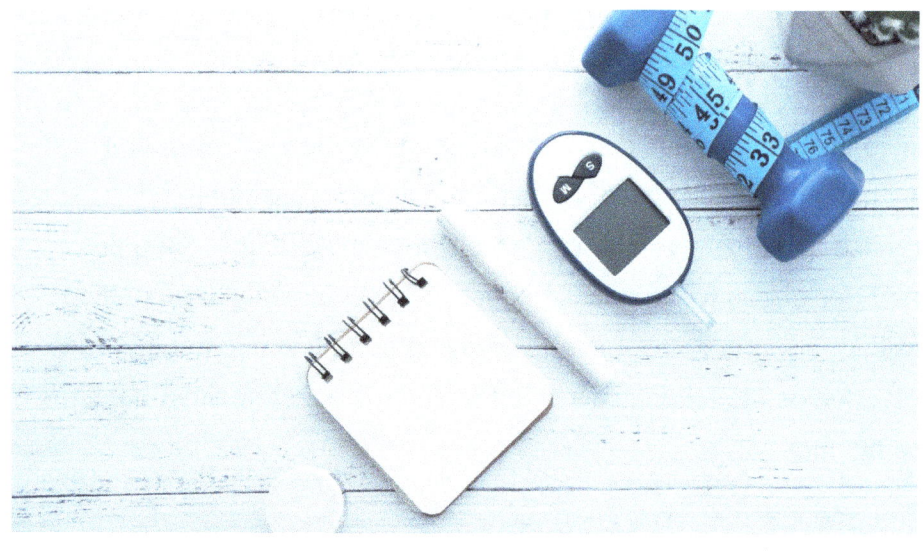

Lesson 1: What is prediabetes?
Lesson 2: Common symptoms and
screening for pre-diabetes

Lesson 1: What is prediabetes?

To understand what prediabetes is and what is happening in your body; first, you must understand what insulin is.

Insulin is a hormone created and released into the bloodstream by the pancreas to redirect blood glucose (sugar) into other areas of the body to be broken down and used as energy.

Insulin is our friend. We want insulin, we need insulin.

Pre-diabetes is a term that describes high blood sugar levels that have not hit the criteria to be considered diabetes. Pre-diabetes is caused by insulin-resistance. Because blood glucose is building up in the bloodstream with nowhere to go; the blood continuously accumulates more and more glucose. This leads to high A1C readings and a pre-diabetes diagnosis.

Insulin-resistance occurs when the cells in your body (usually within the muscles, fat and liver) cannot do its job to release blood glucose from the bloodstream. In other words, the friend with the car is too busy to pick the blood glucose off and bring it to a better environment. So, blood glucose has no other option but to stay in the concentrated environment (aka the bloodstream).

Lesson 2: Common symptoms and screening for pre-diabetes

Unfortunately, prediabetes does not have many symptoms. In fact, many people experience no symptoms at all. Therefore, the only way to know if you are within a pre-diabetic range is to speak to your health care professional and complete a fasting blood glucose test OR a hemoglobin A1C test.

A Few Screening Guidelines for Pre-Diabetes set out by Diabetes Canada says:

- Every person over the age of 35 should be screened for pre-diabetes.
- Every person who has risk-factors for diabetes should be screened earlier than the age of 35 every 3 years.

Common risk-factors include: having high blood pressure, immediate family members living with type 2 diabetes, anyone diagnosed with PCOS (polycystic ovarian syndrome), anyone with a history of gestational diabetes or anyone living with high cholesterol.

Chapter 1: Understanding Pre- Diabetes
Next Steps

Receiving a pre-diabetes diagnosis can be both scary and frustrating. But, I am here to encourage you every step of the way.

I have been where you are. You are not stuck.

Now that you have a deeper understanding of what is going on in your body, it is time to make meaningful changes in your lifestyle to not only reverse prediabetes, but to continue to manage your blood sugar levels throughout your life.

The following chapters will take you through actionable steps that will

help you adopt realistic changes into your life to decrease your blood

sugar levels without feeling overwhelmed.

For more support, contact me directly:

E shaquellefaloncoaching@outlook.com

CHAPTER 2: HEALTHY HABITS TO REVERSE PREDIABETES

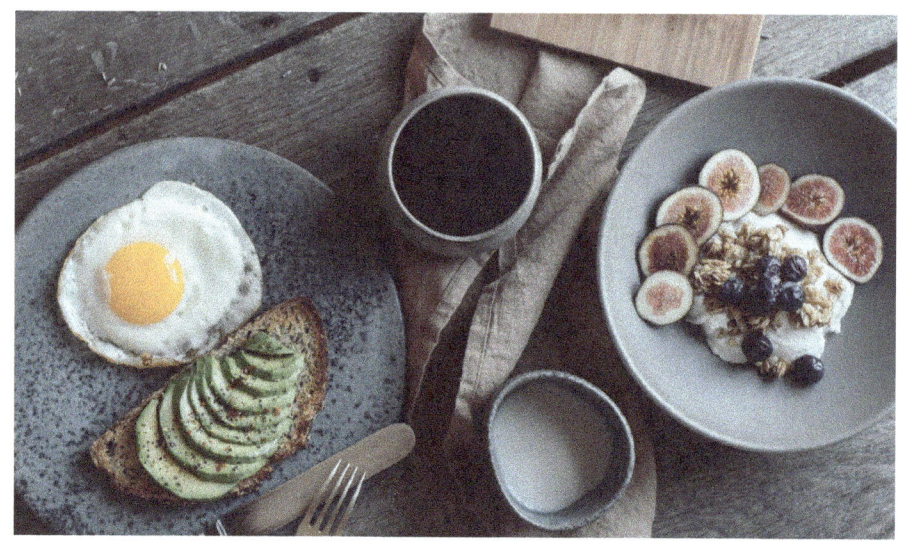

Lesson 1: Dietary adjustments

Lesson 2: Incorporating exercise into your daily routine

Lesson 1: Dietary adjustments

There is no one diet that works for every person; especially when you are aiming to find a long-term solution for blood sugar management. However, the healthy behaviours that have been shown to benefit blood sugar levels include:

- Having regular meals and snacks throughout the day,

- Eating more filling foods (such as high-fibre plant foods and protein)

- introducing more foods that are lower on the glycemic index scale, as well as

- adjusting your mindset about healthy-habits - especially related to food.

1. Eat Regular Meals and Snacks Throughout the Day

According to Diabetes Canada "eating at regular times helps your body control blood sugar levels. It also helps to try to eat about the same amount of food at each meal, especially carbohydrates" (2023). It is also recommended to eat meals no more than 6 hours apart in order to keep your blood sugar levels regulated.

2. Eat Filling Foods Such as High-Fibre Plant Foods and Protein

A high-protein diet has been shown to lower blood glucose in people living with type 2 diabetes and improves overall glucose control. Additionally, plant-based foods include fibre compounds which increase insulin sensitivity, and make insulin more effective at decreasing blood sugar levels.

Lesson 1: Dietary adjustments

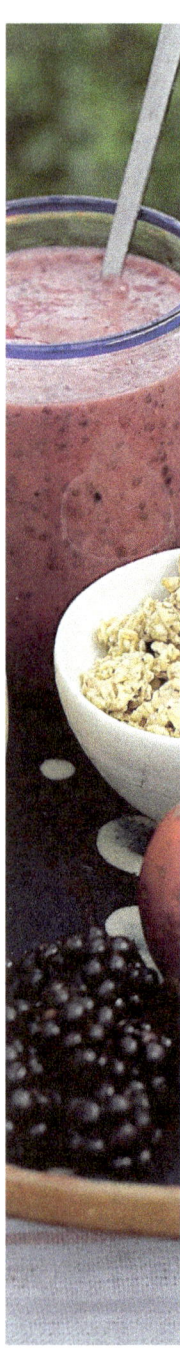

3. Introduce Foods Lower on the Glycemic Index Scale Into Your Diet

The glycemic index is a scale that ranks foods and drinks that have carbohydrates/sugar by how much it raises blood sugar levels after it is consumed. Foods with a high glycemic index increase blood sugar higher and faster than foods with a low glycemic index. Therefore, it is very beneficial to incorporate low glycemic index foods into your meals to manage your blood sugar levels.

4. Adjust Your Mindset About Healthy Habits Especially Related to Food.

Diet culture has affected many people's relationship with food. In the following sections I will refer to a few intuitive eating principles to explain how you can reconnect with your hunger, fullness and satisfaction cues. These three cues are something we are all born with but lose due to social influence surrounding diet, health and weight loss.

The following are dietary changes you can make to approach the change in diet towards more blood sugar friendly foods without feeling like you're stuck in a rigid diet.

- **Reject Diet Mentality:**

  Unlearn the "weight loss and health" tips that created the idea that certain foods are bad for you and others are good for you. Instead, recognize the different nutritional value and glycemic index each food contains and trial different combinations of these foods to discover what works best for you (and your blood sugar levels).

- **Challenge the Food Police:**

  The food police is the voice in your head that makes you feel "guilty" for eating specific foods. When searching for long-term solutions for your health, it is important to honour what your body wants and needs. Therefore, there is no need to feel guilty about your choices and enter a loop of strict dieting, not following the diet and then feeling guilty again.

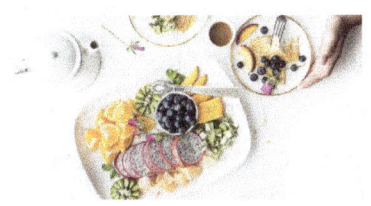

- **Discover the Satisfaction Factor:**

    Let's be honest, eating can provide a source of pleasure (and if you're reading this right now saying no it doesn't… I don't believe you). By fighting yourself to refrain from enjoying a specific meal, you are not allowing yourself to satisfy the mental and emotional component of eating. Which could allow for binge-ing habits in the future as a way to achieve the satisfaction you were looking for.

- **Feel Your Fullness:**

    It is important to acknowledge when you are feeling full. It is a signal from your body telling you it is physically satisfied. And, research shows this can allow for improvements in A1C levels in the long run.

- **Cope with Your Emotions with Kindness:**

    Emotional eating is a common pattern that people fall into. Coping with your emotions in a positive way allows you to acknowledge when emotional eating is occurring and begin strategies to cope with your emotions in a more effective way. Emotional eating could affect blood sugar control because one tends to look for foods that increase the "happy hormone" quickly. Usually these go-to, happy hormone foods are filled with sugar (which will negatively affect your blood sugar levels).

Lesson 2: Incorporating exercise into your daily routine

Research has shown that adding bouts of physical activity within your day decreases your chances of developing type 2 diabetes. If you are contemplating if your daily walks or stretches are worth the effort, they are! Remember to make exercise fun by adding it in your day when you can.

Effective exercise does not have to include pushing so hard in the gym that you almost throw up. Search for an exercise option that you enjoy. Once you find something you enjoy it will motivate you to participate in exercise more regularly; which will help you manage your blood sugar levels.

It took me years to commit to a workout plan. It took even longer for me to realize that it's okay to switch your exercise plan when necessary and still stay consistent in your health goals.

Below I dive into ways to add exercise into your life when a rigid workout routine is just not doing it for you. I want you to know that it is perfectly okay and effective to find ways to get active outside of the gym.

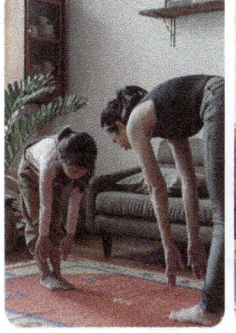 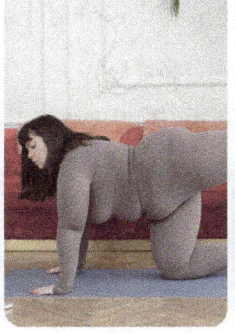 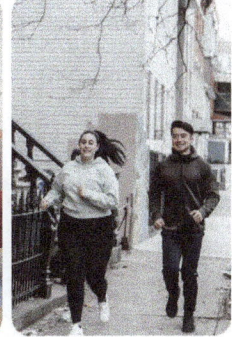

Try the following tips below to gradually increase exercise in your day over time. You will see long-term results with consistency in routine.

- **Active transportation/Improve your daily commute:** Find opportunities in your day to fit exercise in on your commute. For every person this may look different. If you drive to work could you find a parking spot a block away and walk the rest? Is it possible to cycle to work? Or bus part-way and walk the rest? Active transportation provides long term health benefits and improves blood sugar levels.
- **Use Your Breaks Wisely:** Similar to active transportation, fit movement into your breaks while at work or school. This tip can be especially useful if you are working from home or at a desk. Take a walk around the block on your coffee break, walk up and down your hallway while in phone meetings, take a walking lunch break and eat outside, or take a 3–5 minute stretch break every few hours at work. A study done in 2016 demonstrates that taking active breaks throughout the day decreases employees' physical ailments in the long-run, reduces stress and increases productivity.
- **Schedule Exercise in as a Non-Negotiable Meeting:** Having a regular exercise routine is important in order to see both short and long term benefits in all dimensions of wellness. By scheduling in your exercise and making it a non-negotiable you are setting yourself for long-term success.

It is easy for many of us to skip our workouts to attend a last-minute work meeting, run errands or other reasons. Eliminate the possibility of skipping your workout by scheduling it in as a mandatory meeting for yourself to attend.

For some people, committing to a structured exercise routine is most beneficial. There are many ways to go about this but again, joyful movement is top priority for long term adherence to a plan. Here are ideas for you to access more structured fitness regimes.

1. **Join a local gym:**

   - Joining a local gym can be helpful for focusing on your workout. When working out at home or even outdoors there could be distractions that deter you from completing your routine.

   - For more support on joining a gym to help manage your blood sugar levels, please see the free exercise templates in the resources section.

2. **Connect with an exercise professional.**

   - Speak to a personal trainer, kinesiologist or coach to create a personalized exercise plan and support you in the gym. The benefits of meeting with an certified exercise professional includes: structured workouts that suit your needs and interests, ongoing support and motivation to hit your goals.

   - For structured support from me, a Registered Kinesiologist, send me an email at: **shaquellefaloncoaching@outlook.com**

3. **Join an on-demand exercise platform:**
   - There are a variety of online platforms that provide on-demand workouts. Enjoy a structured workout in the comfort of your own home if working out in the gym doesn't feel right for you.
   - Send an email to shaquellefaloncoaching@outlook.com for more information on how to join!

4. **Join a local group fitness studio:**
   - Group fitness classes may be a great option for you if you are looking to join an in-person community for structured exercise. It will allow you to connect with like-minded individuals, stay accountable to regular exercise sessions and decrease the stress around figuring out what to do in the gym.
   - Search your area for a group fitness studio you feel comfortable in. Below you will see a couple group fitness studios I recommend due to their positive outlook on health and welcoming environment.

     - **In Toronto, ON: SisterFit Toronto**
     - **In Winnipeg, MB: Blue Sky Fitness**

5. **Find a virtual exercise platform that suits your needs:**
   - If you are looking to workout live with an instructor but are not ready to join an in-person gym, search online for a virtual platform that provides live classes. Below I have mentioned a wonderful community that provides live online classes.
     - **Body Positive Fitness**

Chapter 2: Healthy Habits to Reverse Prediabetes

Next Steps

There are a variety of options to consider when making changes to your current nutrition and exercise routine. My biggest piece of advice to you is to make changes **one step at a time.**

If you are unsure of where to start, I recommend making a list of the current habits that you take part in that you enjoy and would like to continue with as well as make a list of the habits you would like to improve on.

Once your list is complete, number the habits you would like to improve on from 1-10 (1 being the least scary habit to change and 10 being the scariest/hardest habit to change).

Then, use the tools found in this chapter to move through changing each habit at a time.

For more support, contact me directly:

shaquellefaloncoaching@outlook.com

CHAPTER 3: TAKING CONTROL OF YOUR HEALTH

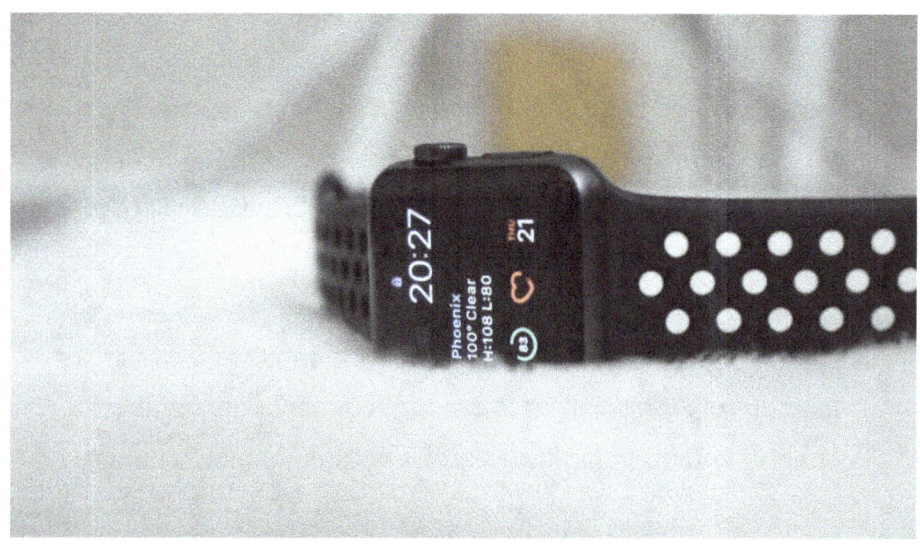

Lesson 1: Healthy Habits

Lesson 2: Going Beyond Diet and Exercise

Lesson 1: Healthy Habits

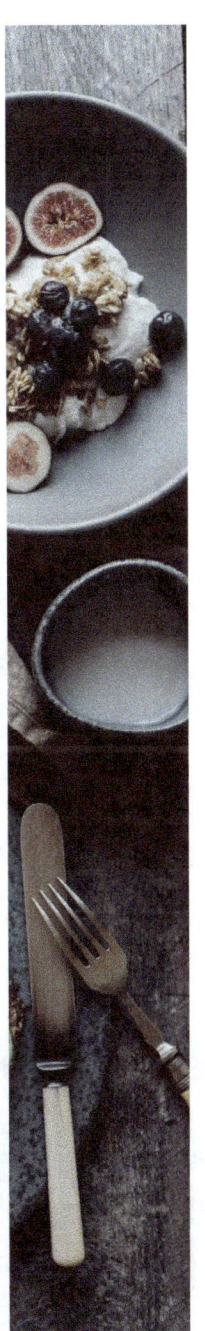

There have been many times I have started a new "healthy" habit and stopped not too long after.

Sometimes it's not easy to start new routines and keep up with them. But, there are ways to see success when creating a new routine for a new habit.

Type 2 diabetes, and any other condition related to insulin-resistance, can have long-term effects on your body. So, it is best to skip the fad diets and take a different approach to managing your blood sugar levels to reverse your prediabetes diagnosis. Habit-stacking may be an approach that works for you.

Habit-stacking is a strategy used to build habits through grouping different activities together. The reason why habit-stacking works so well in relation to health goals is because you eliminate the excuse of having "no time".

With this method, you add the new healthy habits you're trying to gain to daily habits you already perform. The key to being successful here is to treat the daily habit and new habit as one. This will eliminate feeling overwhelmed about completing too much at once or feeling like you don't have enough time to complete your new habits.

Here are five steps for you to take to successfully complete habit-stacking.

Use 5 Minute Timers

No matter what habit you are trying to build, I recommend setting a timer for 5 minutes to do it. Setting a five-minute timer will allow you to focus on the new task and commit to spending time towards participating in the specific habit.

One example of this could be setting a 5 minute timer as soon as you get out of bed to stretch as you scroll through social media in the morning. Scrolling on social media as soon as you wake up is the "habit" you already participate in daily, so, we are leveraging this five-minutes you already have set in your day to adopt a new healthy-habit.

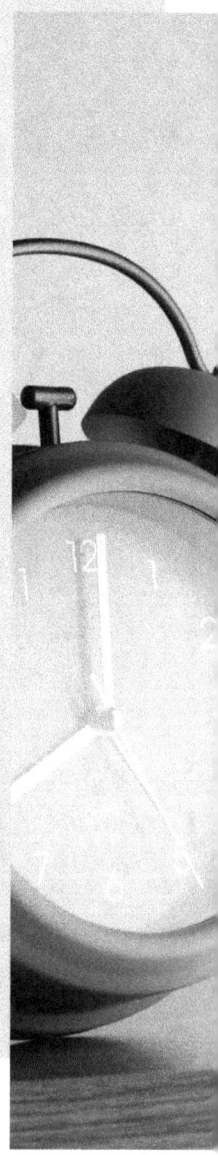

Schedule Intentional Time Into Your Day

Put your specific healthy-habit into your calendar for the day. This will add accountability for you and an extra reminder for you to get your tasks done. Make sure you get specific with this and pick a time and location for the task to be done every day.

An example of this is, every morning when you get into the office from work you start the day off by checking your emails. Since checking your emails first is already a daily task you participate in, add drinking at least one full glass of water before you switch tasks. Now, you've added the new task to a habit you already participate in daily with a specific time and place specified.

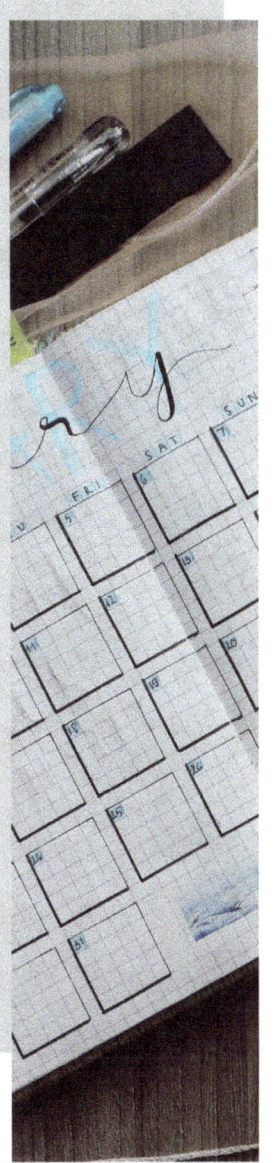

Choose Your Method For Reminders

Having alarms on your phone and calendar reminders are great. But, you want to have reminders in place to keep on top of your habits separate from your devices. You want to lean into your five senses to create more of an almost "automatic" response for you to complete your task.

For example, every time you open the fridge for a snack, you do 5 squats. Opening the fridge is a habit you do daily, so, as a reminder for you to participate in exercise without you having to think about it. This habit will remind you to exercise.

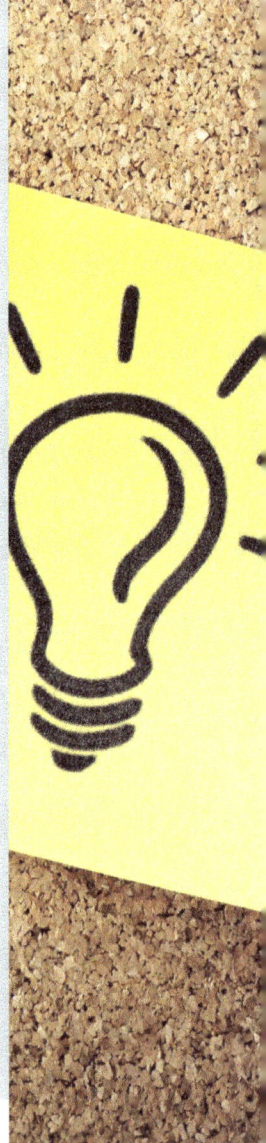

Stay Accountable

Having an external cue or system in place to keep you accountable is one of the best ways to successfully create new healthy habits. Consider meeting with a friendly weekly or monthly to chat about your goals and keep track of how you are doing.

Another idea is to find an accountability buddy that you check in with every day. It is helpful to be checking in with someone regularly who has similar goals as you to keep you both motivated. Another option is to invest in a coach or personal trainer. These high-level professionals can not only keep you accountable but push you to become even better than you thought!

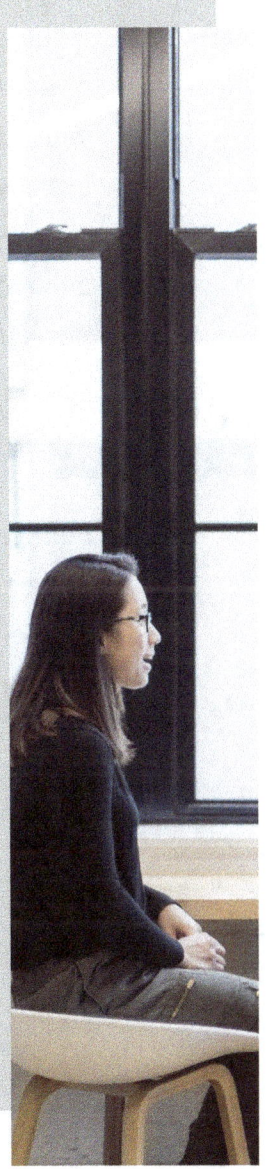

Take it One Habit At a Time

The biggest mistake people make after receiving a scary diagnosis is to try to change everything at once. It's that all-or-nothing mindset that ends up getting you stuck in the off-and-on dieting cycle without seeing long-term results. After working with both prediabetes and type 2 diabetes clientele for over the last few years I have seen drastic long-term changes due to taking everything one step at a time!

Furthermore, <u>research</u> shows that off-and-on dieting cycles are more harmful for the body than not; especially if you are living with type 2 diabetes.

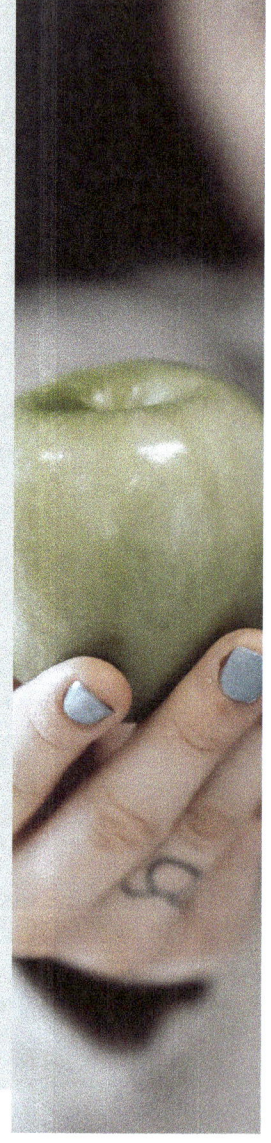

Here is a list of habit-stacking practices you can use to drop your blood sugar levels.

- Use the first 5–10 minutes of your lunch break at work to take a walk.
- Drink one glass of water with breakfast in the morning.
- Do 5 squats every time you open TikTok or Instagram.
- Do alternating lunges while you brush your teeth.
- Eat a piece of fruit or a vegetable whenever you eat a piece of chocolate.
- Complete a 5 minute stretch right before you get into bed for the night.

When first starting to habit-stack it can feel a bit overwhelming. So, take it one habit at a time and one task at a time. Slow and consistent efforts towards your healthy habits is the best way to see long term changes in your A1C levels.

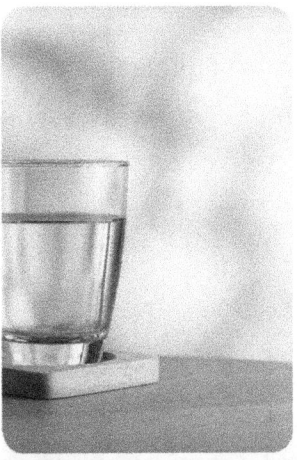

Lesson 2: Going Beyond Diet and Exercise

There are many factors to consider when managing your blood sugar levels that extend further than diet and exercise. Other aspects of your health you should be mindful of is sleep, stress and mental health.

1. **The Importance of Sleep**

    - Sleep is a staple part of balancing your overall well-being. But, with balancing all the demands of life such as school, work, family, recreation and more; sleep is commonly put on the back-burner. A loss of sleep has been <u>shown</u> to cause impairments in glucose metabolism as well as contribute to insulin resistance.

    - <u>Studies</u> show that 1 in 5 Canadian adults under the age of 65 get less than 7 hours of sleep per night. Less than 7 hours of sleep per night can cause an increase in appetite, makes you reach for more high-carb foods (the body's way of gaining fast energy), raise blood pressure, decrease immune function and reduce how full you feel after meals.

Did you know if you get less than 7 hours of sleep per night your blood sugar levels will be harder to manage?

Here are a few tips to help you get a more restful sleep and improve your blood sugar management:

- Put down the electronics and turn off the TV one hour before bed.
- Keep your bedroom dark with blackout curtains and all lamps off.
- Exercise throughout the day rather than right before bed. Avoid evening caffeine as that can keep the body's energy up and make it more difficult to fall asleep.
- Create a bedtime routine to help yourself relax.
- Don't eat a heavy meal right before bed (a snack is totally fine).

2. Stress Management

Stress in the body can lead to increased blood glucose and an insensitivity to insulin production in the long run. Therefore, it is important to include regular stress management practices into your lifestyle to manage your stress.

A common method used to manage stress is following the 4 "A's".

AVOID   **ALTAR**

ADAPT   **ACCEPT**

AVOID

Not all stressors in life are avoidable. But, there are environmental stressors that can arise and be benefitted by avoidance.
For example, if you become stressed while scrolling through social media or any online platform it may be best to walk away from the phone for some time and avoid those platforms. Similarly, if you are in a physical environment

ALTAR

Some stressors are part of our day-to-day routines. For example, you may have a jam-packed day full of meetings and commitments; and this type of schedule causes some levels of anxiety. Two important steps to take in this situation would be to communicate your emotions and consider altering your schedule to meet your comfort level.

ADAPT

In life, situations come up where you are not able to avoid or adjust to suit your personal needs. So, adapting to the situation may be the only option. Try to reframe the seemingly stressful situation. Changing how you look at and approach a situation can help relieve stress and even help you look at the situation in a positive light.

ACCEPT

It is important to accept that stress can come from a variety of situations and could be unchangeable. Move through life acknowledging your power and understanding what IS in your control, and always keep your eyes open for the opportunities that may lie in any given situation.

My number one piece of advice if you are dealing with mental health struggles is to contact a mental health professional. Seeking professional help can be uncomfortable and overwhelming but, once you find the right person to work with — your healing process will be game-changing.

Below is a list of mental health professionals you can reach out to for virtual support:

- Elysia Bronson, Registered Clinical Counsellor
  www.thewoodscounselling.com
- Dr. Sam Clouthier, Naturopathic Doctor
  www.junipernaturopathic.com
- Miranda Klimowski, Registered Psychotherapist
  mirandaklimowskicounselling@gmail.com
- Jasmine Tsang, Registered Psychotherapist (Qualifying)
  hello@reflectionspsychotherapy.ca

Chapter 3: Taking Control of Your Health
Next Steps

When it comes to reversing your blood sugar levels it is imperative that you take into account all aspects of your wellness.

The body is a complex structure that needs to be acknowledge holistically in order to find balance.

Just like I've said many times before in this book; take each change one step at a time.

You will find your balance.

For more support, contact me directly:

E shaquellefaloncoaching@outlook.com

Conclusion

A healthy lifestyle is a life-long journey. It will ebb and flow and change with different seasons of life. Please remember to be gentle with yourself and take on your healthy changes one habit at a time.

Once you have completed the e-book; I encourage you to go through it again, chapter-by-chapter, with one habit you are working on changing at a time. With each habit you adjust, you will understand and internalize the process - making you more comfortable in changing the scarier habits. For more support please contact me. I am always happy to help.

For more support, contact me directly:

✉ shaquellefaloncoaching@outlook.com
Instagram: @shaquellefaloncoaching
Facebook Group: "Shaq's Wellness Community"

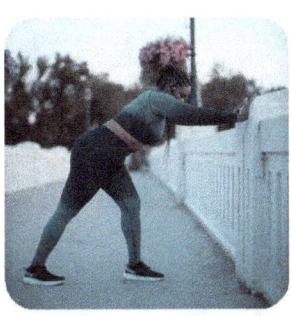

Glossary

Glycemic Index - The glycemic index is a scale that ranks foods and drinks that have carbohydrates/sugar by how much it raises blood sugar levels after it is consumed.

Intuitive Eating - A personal health journey where you get to reconnect with your hunger, fullness and satisfaction cues.

Habit Stacking - a strategy used to build habits through grouping different activities together.

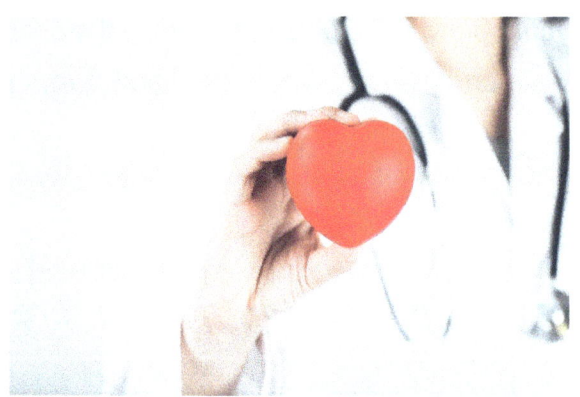

RESOURCES

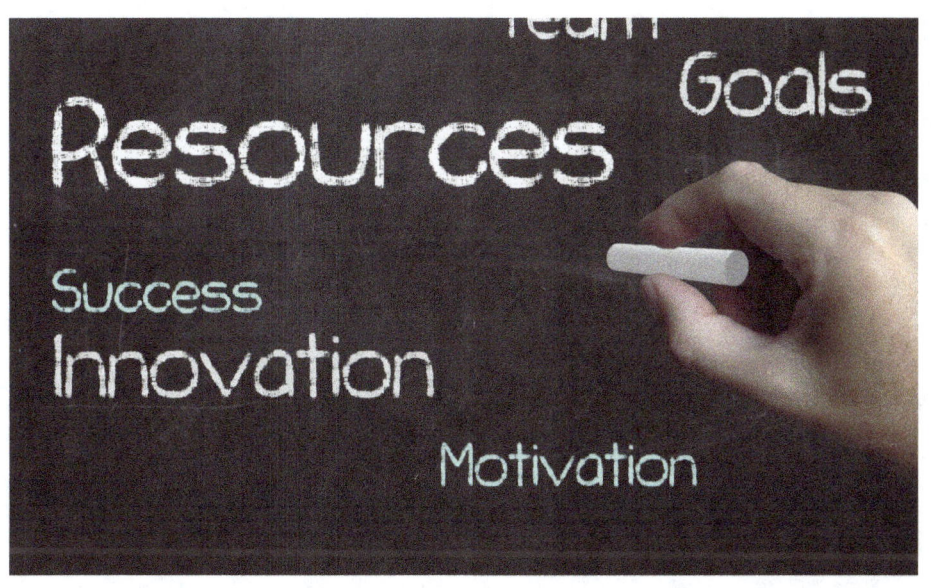

36-39: Glycemic Index Charts (Diabetes Canada)

40-43: Free Workouts

Glycemic Index Food Guide

The glycemic index (GI) is a scale that ranks a carbohydrate-containing food or drink by how much it raises blood sugar levels after it is eaten or drank. Foods with a high GI increase blood sugar higher and faster than foods with a low GI.

There are three GI categories:

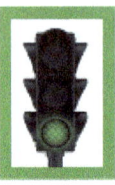  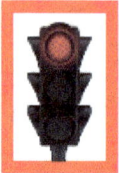

Green = Go
Low GI (55 or less) Choose Most Often

Yellow = Caution
Medium GI (56 to 69) Choose Less Often

Red = Stop and think
High GI (70 or more) Choose Least Often

Foods in the high GI category can be swapped with foods in the medium and/or low GI category to lower GI.

A low GI diet may help you:

- decrease risk of type 2 diabetes and its complications
- decrease risk of heart disease and stroke
- feel full longer
- maintain or lose weight

Try these meal planning ideas to lower meal GI:

- Cook your pasta al dente (firm). Check your pasta package instructions for cooking time.
- Make fruits and milk part of your meal plate (Figure 1). These foods often have a low GI and make a healthy dessert.
- Try lower GI grains, such as barley and bulgur.
- Pulses can be grains and starches or meat and alternatives. Swap half of your higher GI starch food serving with beans, lentils or chickpeas. For example, instead of having 1 cup of cooked short grain rice, have ½ cup of cooked rice mixed with ½ cup of black beans.

Diabetes Canada recommends choosing lower GI foods and drinks more often to help control blood sugar.

Work with your Registered Dietitian to add foods and drinks to your lists, create action plans that include choosing lower GI foods, adapt your favourite recipes, and find ways to swap/substitute low GI foods into your meal plan.

Checking your blood sugar before, and 2 hours after, a meal is the best way to know how your body handles certain foods and drinks.

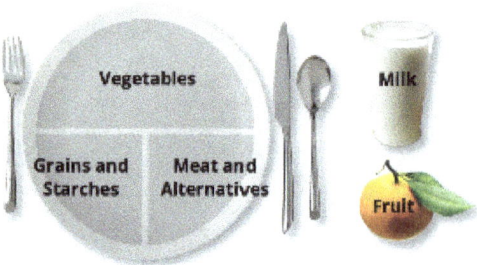

Figure 1: The Plate Method. Using a standard dinner plate, follow this model to control your portion sizes. www.diabetes.ca/mealplanning

Some carbohydrate-containing foods and drinks have so little carbohydrate that they do not have a GI value. This does not mean they cannot be included as part of a healthy diet. Examples include green vegetables, lemons, and some low-carbohydrate drinks. Diabetes Canada calls these foods and drinks "free" because they do not impact the blood sugar of people living with diabetes. You can put free foods in the green category, but they do not have a GI and have not been included in the food lists.

 Items with this symbol are "sometimes foods" (foods and drinks eaten only on occasion)

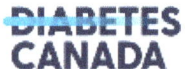

Grains and Starches

Low Glycemic Index (55 or less) Choose Most Often	Medium Glycemic Index (56 to 69) Choose Less Often	High Glycemic Index (70 or more) Choose Least Often
Breads: Heavy Mixed Grain Breads Spelt Bread Sourdough Bread Tortilla (Whole Grain) **Cereal:** All-Bran™ Cereal All-Bran Buds™ With Psyllium Cereal Oat Bran Oats (Steel Cut) **Grains:** Barley Bulgur Mung Bean Noodles Pasta (Al Dente, Firm) Pulse Flours Quinoa Rice (Converted, Parboiled) **Other:** Peas Popcorn Sweet Potato Winter Squash	**Breads:** Chapati (White, Whole Wheat) Flaxseed/Linseed Bread Pita Bread (White, Whole Wheat) Pumpernickel Bread Roti (White, Whole Wheat) Rye Bread (Light, Dark, Whole Grain) Stone Ground Whole Wheat Bread Whole Grain Wheat Bread **Cereal:** Cream of Wheat™ (Regular) Oats (Instant) Oats (Large Flake) Oats (Quick) **Grains:** Basmati Rice Brown Rice Cornmeal Couscous (Regular, Whole Wheat) Rice Noodles White Rice (Short, Long Grain) Wild Rice **Other:** Beets* Corn French Fries ⚠ Parsnip Potato (Red, White, Cooled) Rye Crisp Crackers (e.g. Ryvita Rye Crispbread™) Stoned Wheat Thins™ Crackers	**Breads:** Bread (White, Whole Wheat) Naan (White, Whole Wheat) **Cereal:** All-Bran Flakes™ Cereal Corn Flakes™ Cereal Cream of Wheat™ (Instant) Puffed Wheat Cereal Rice Krispies™ Cereal Special K™ Cereal **Grains:** Jasmine Rice Millet Sticky Rice White Rice (Instant) **Other:** Carrots* Potato (Instant Mashed) Potato (Red, White, Hot) Pretzels Rice Cakes Soda Crackers
Additional foods: 1. 2. 3.	**Additional foods:** 1. 2. 3.	**Additional foods:** 1. 2. 3.

* Most starchy/sweet vegetables (e.g. peas, parsnip, winter squash) provide 15 g or more carbohydrate per 1 cup serving. Beets and carrots often provide less than 15 g carbohydrate per serving (marked above with *). Most non-starchy (or free) vegetables (e.g. tomato and lettuce) have not been assigned a GI because they have very little carbohydrate and have very little effect on blood sugar.

Fruits

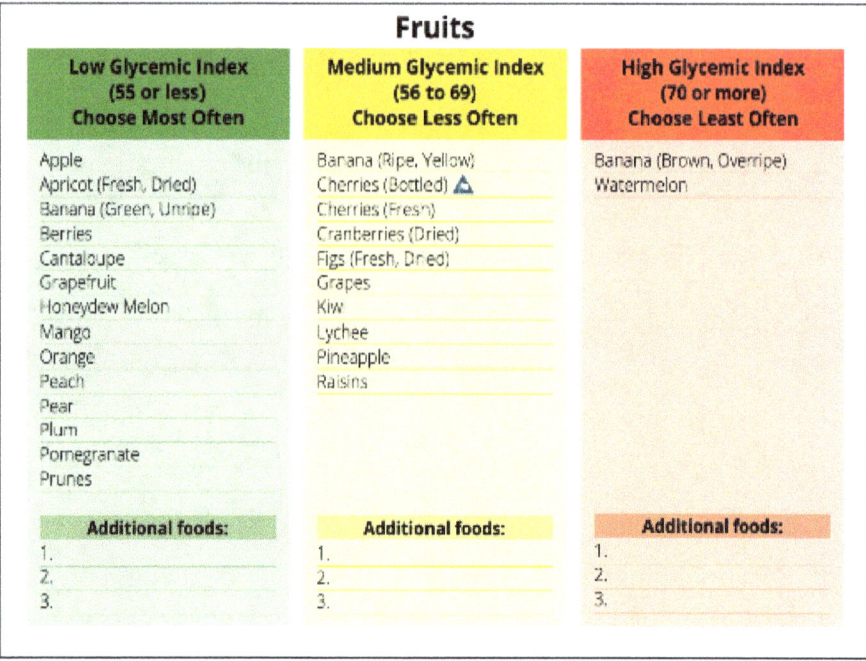

Low Glycemic Index (55 or less) **Choose Most Often**	Medium Glycemic Index (56 to 69) **Choose Less Often**	High Glycemic Index (70 or more) **Choose Least Often**
Apple	Banana (Ripe, Yellow)	Banana (Brown, Overripe)
Apricot (Fresh, Dried)	Cherries (Bottled) ▲	Watermelon
Banana (Green, Unripe)	Cherries (Fresh)	
Berries	Cranberries (Dried)	
Cantaloupe	Figs (Fresh, Dried)	
Grapefruit	Grapes	
Honeydew Melon	Kiwi	
Mango	Lychee	
Orange	Pineapple	
Peach	Raisins	
Pear		
Plum		
Pomegranate		
Prunes		
Additional foods:	**Additional foods:**	**Additional foods:**
1.	1.	1.
2.	2.	2.
3.	3.	3.

Some fruits have not been assigned a GI because they contain less than 15 g of available carbohydrate per serving (e.g. lemon and lime).

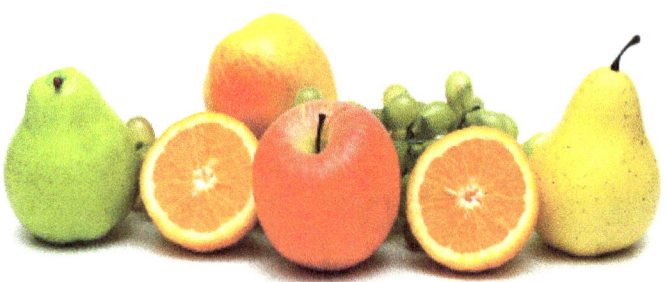

Many fruits and vegetables fall in the
low or medium GI categories.

Milk, Alternatives and Other Beverages

Low Glycemic Index (55 or less) Choose Most Often	Medium Glycemic Index (56 to 69) Choose Less Often	High Glycemic Index (70 or more) Choose Least Often
Almond Milk Cow Milk (Skim, 1%, 2%, Whole) Frozen Yogurt △ Greek Yogurt Soy Milk Yogurt (Skim, 1%, 2%, Whole)		Rice Milk
Additional foods: 1. 2. 3.	**Additional foods:** 1. 2. 3.	**Additional foods:** 1. 2. 3.

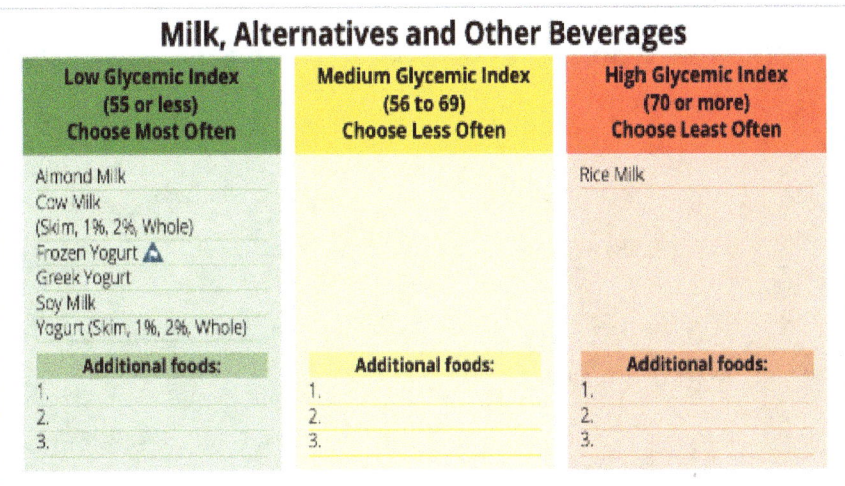

Milk, alternatives, and other beverages listed include flavoured (e.g. chocolate), sweetened and unsweetened varieties.

Meat and Alternatives

Low Glycemic Index (55 or less) Choose Most Often	Medium Glycemic Index (56 to 69) Choose Less Often	High Glycemic Index (70 or more) Choose Least Often
Baked Beans Chickpeas Kidney Beans Lentils Mung Beans Romano Beans Soybeans/Edamame Split Peas	Lentil Soup (ready-made) Split Pea Soup (ready-made)	
Additional foods: 1. 2. 3.	**Additional foods:** 1. 2. 3.	**Additional foods:** 1. 2. 3.

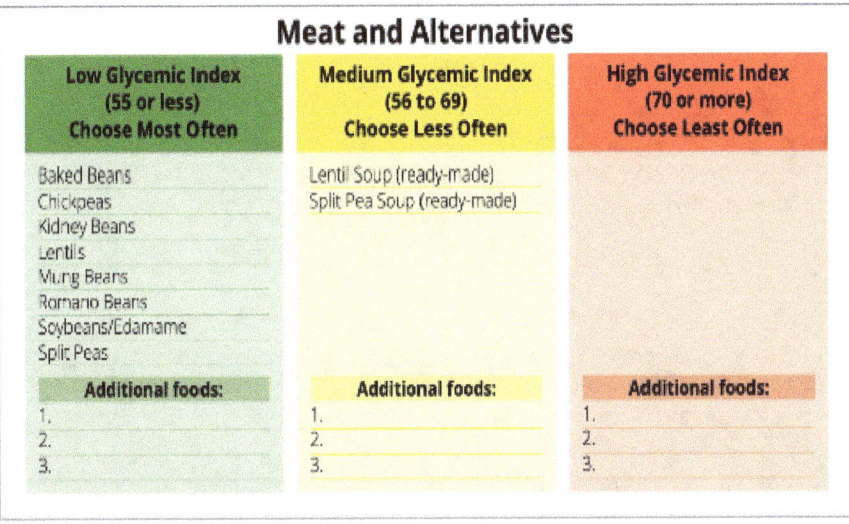

Meat, poultry and fish do not have a GI because they do not contain carbohydrate. When ½ cup or more of pulses are eaten, they can be included in the Grains and Starches food group or the Meats and Alternatives group.

Diabetes Canada is making the invisible epidemic of diabetes visible and urgent. Eleven million Canadians have diabetes or prediabetes. Now is the time to End Diabetes - its health impacts, as well as the blame, shame and misinformation associated with it. Diabetes Canada partners with Canadians to End Diabetes through education and support services, resources for health-care professionals, advocacy to governments, schools and workplaces, and funding research to improve treatments and find a cure.

This document reflects the *Canadian Diabetes Association 2013 Clinical Practice Guidelines for the Prevention and Management of Diabetes in Canada* © 2013 The Canadian Diabetes Association. The Canadian Diabetes Association is the registered owner of the name Diabetes Canada. 115009 02/18

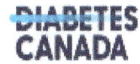

Beginner Strength Training

FOR THE GYM

WARM UP

Exercise	Exercise
2x30secs Cat-Cows	2x30secs Arm Circles
2x30secs Squats	2x30secs Lateral Lunges

STRENGTH TRAINING

Exercise	Set	Rep	Heart Rate
Goblet Reverse Lunges	2	10-12	
Seated Leg Curls	2	10-12	
Glute Bridges	2	10-12	
Bent-Over Rows	2	10-12	
Chest Flys	2	10-12	
Hammer Curl and Shoulder Press	2	10-12	
Triceps Kickbacks	2	10-12	
Bicycle Crunches	2	10	

CARDIO

Exercise	Set	Rep	Heart Rate
Elliptical or Treadmill	1	15-20 mins	

Beginner Strength Training

FOR HOME

WARM UP

Exercise

2x30secs Squats

2x30secs Arm Circles

2x30secs Lateral Lunges

2x30secs Cat-Cows

STRENGTH TRAINING

Exercise	Set	Rep	Heart Rate
Squats	2	10-12	
Good Mornings	2	10-12	
Jumping Jacks	2	10-12	
Glute Bridges	2	10-12	
Supermans	2	10-12	
Kneeling Push Ups	2	10-12	
Crunches	2	10-12	

NOTES

Intermediate Strength Training

FOR THE GYM

WARM UP

Exercise

2x30secs Squats   2x30secs Arm Circles

2x30secs Lateral Lunges   2x30secs Cat-Cows

STRENGTH TRAINING

Exercise	Set	Reps	Heart Rate
Goblet Squats	3	10-12	
Romanian Deadlifts	3	10-12	
Seated Rows	3	10-12	
Chest Flys	3	10-12	
Hammer Curl and Shoulder Press	3	10-12	
Triceps Kickbacks	3	10-12	
Side Plank	3	45 secs	
Bicycle Crunches	3	45 secs	

CARDIO

Exercise	Set	Reps	Heart Rate
Elliptical or Stationary Bike	1	15-20 mins	

Intermediate Strength Training

FOR HOME

WARM UP

Exercise

2x30secs Squats	2x30secs Arm Circles
2x30secs Lateral Lunges	2x30secs Cat-Cows

STRENGTH TRAINING

Exercise	Set	Rep	Heart Rate
Walking Lunges	3	10-12	
Jumping Jacks	3	15-20	
Good Mornings	3	10-12	
Supermans	3	15-20	
Push Ups	3	10-12	
Mountain Climbers	3	45 secs	
Glute Bridges	3	15-20	
Bicycle Crunches	3	45 secs	

NOTES

References

https://journals.sagepub.com/doi/full/10.1177/2165079916653416

https://journals.sagepub.com/doi/10.1177/1358863X19850316?
url_ver=Z39.88-
2003&rfr_id=ori:rid:crossref.org&rfr_dat=cr_pub%20%200pubmed

https://www.sciencedirect.com/science/article/abs/pii/S009174
3515001164?via%3Dihub=&source=post_page-----ff8d2ed5f64f----

https://pubmed.ncbi.nlm.nih.gov/37039787/

https://www.statcan.gc.ca/o1/en/plus/581-world-sleep-day?
source=post_page   eec7fac4bf61

https://pubmed.ncbi.nlm.nih.gov/34779405/

https://www.ncbi.nlm.nih.gov/pmc/articles/PMC2084401/?
source=post_page   eec7fac4bf61

https://www.diabetes.ca/

https://pubmed.ncbi.nlm.nih.gov/14522731/

https://journals.sagepub.com/doi/full/10.1177/2165079916653416

https://link.springer.com/article/10.1007/BF01219783

https://www.ncbi.nlm.nih.gov/pmc/articles/PMC2084401/

https://www.statcan.gc.ca/o1/en/plus/581-world-sleep-day

https://www.ncbi.nlm.nih.gov/pmc/articles/PMC9561544/#:~:text
=Blood%20sugar%20levels%20may%20rise,regulation%20of%20the
se%20stress%20hormones.

www.ingramcontent.com/pod-product-compliance
Lightning Source LLC
Chambersburg PA
CBHW070344290526
45791CB00003B/1463